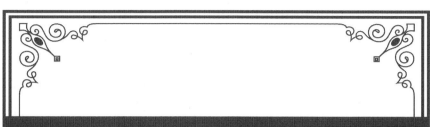

# THANK YOU
*for your purchase*

★ ★ **WE HOPE YOU ENJOY THIS BOOK** ★ ★

All feedback is greatly appreciated as it lets us know how we are doing!

For any inquiries please feel free to email us at:
**Contact@mgpublish.com**

## WANT A FREEBIE?!

Signup for a free gift at:

**Mgpublish.com/free-download**

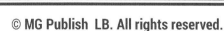

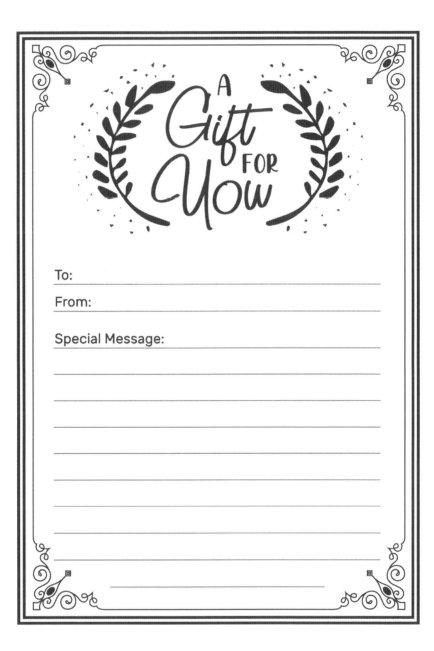

A Gift FOR You

To:

From:

Special Message:

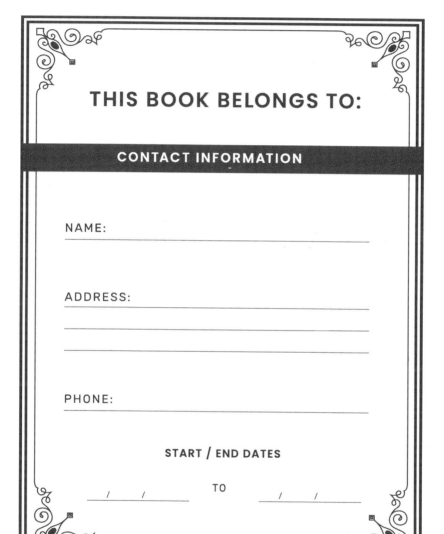

# THIS BOOK BELONGS TO:

## CONTACT INFORMATION

NAME: _____

ADDRESS: _____

_____

_____

PHONE: _____

### START / END DATES

_____ / _____ / _____  TO  _____ / _____ / _____

# MEDICAL PROFILE

| | |
|---|---|
| **NAME** | |
| **DATE OF BIRTH** | **BLOOD TYPE** |

| DRUG ALLERGIES | FOOD ALLERGIES |
|---|---|
| ○ | ○ |
| ○ | ○ |
| ○ | ○ |
| ○ | ○ |
| ○ | ○ |
| ○ | ○ |
| ○ | ○ |

## MEDICAL HISTORY

## MEDICATION

# FAMILY HEALTH HISTORY

|  | FATHER | MOTHER | GRAND PARENTS (F) | GRAND PARENTS (M) |
|---|---|---|---|---|
| HEART DISEASE | O | O | O | O |
| CANCER | O | O | O | O |
| DIABETES | O | O | O | O |
| LIVER DISEASE | O | O | O | O |
| STROKE | O | O | O | O |
| THYROID (H/L) | O | O | O | O |
| DEPRESSION / SUICIDE | O | O | O | O |
| EPILEPSY | O | O | O | O |
| KIDNEY DISEASE | O | O | O | O |
|  | O | O | O | O |
|  | O | O | O | O |
|  | O | O | O | O |
|  | O | O | O | O |
|  | O | O | O | O |

## PHYSICIANS

| NAME | SPECIALITY | ADDRESS | PHONE |
|---|---|---|---|
|  |  |  |  |
|  |  |  |  |
|  |  |  |  |
|  |  |  |  |
|  |  |  |  |
|  |  |  |  |
|  |  |  |  |

## NOTES

# MEDICAL INSURANCE INFO

| | |
|---|---|
| NAME | |
| PROVIDER | |
| POLICY NUMBER | |
| POLICY TYPE | |
| ADDRESS | |
| PHONE NUMBER | EMAIL |
| NOTES | |

| | |
|---|---|
| NAME | |
| PROVIDER | |
| POLICY NUMBER | |
| POLICY TYPE | |
| ADDRESS | |
| PHONE NUMBER | EMAIL |
| NOTES | |

| | |
|---|---|
| NAME | |
| PROVIDER | |
| POLICY NUMBER | |
| POLICY TYPE | |
| ADDRESS | |
| PHONE NUMBER | EMAIL |
| NOTES | |

# MEDICAL INSURANCE INFO

| | |
|---|---|
| **NAME** | |
| **PROVIDER** | |
| **POLICY NUMBER** | |
| **POLICY TYPE** | |
| **ADDRESS** | |
| **PHONE NUMBER** | **EMAIL** |
| **NOTES** | |

| | |
|---|---|
| **NAME** | |
| **PROVIDER** | |
| **POLICY NUMBER** | |
| **POLICY TYPE** | |
| **ADDRESS** | |
| **PHONE NUMBER** | **EMAIL** |
| **NOTES** | |

| | |
|---|---|
| **NAME** | |
| **PROVIDER** | |
| **POLICY NUMBER** | |
| **POLICY TYPE** | |
| **ADDRESS** | |
| **PHONE NUMBER** | **EMAIL** |
| **NOTES** | |

# ILLNESS RECORD

| DATE | DIAGNOSIS | MEDICATION | DOCTOR |
|------|-----------|------------|--------|
|      |           |            |        |
|      |           |            |        |
|      |           |            |        |
|      |           |            |        |
|      |           |            |        |
|      |           |            |        |
|      |           |            |        |
|      |           |            |        |
|      |           |            |        |
|      |           |            |        |
|      |           |            |        |
|      |           |            |        |
|      |           |            |        |
|      |           |            |        |
|      |           |            |        |
|      |           |            |        |
|      |           |            |        |
|      |           |            |        |
|      |           |            |        |
|      |           |            |        |
|      |           |            |        |
|      |           |            |        |
|      |           |            |        |
|      |           |            |        |
|      |           |            |        |
|      |           |            |        |
|      |           |            |        |
|      |           |            |        |
|      |           |            |        |
|      |           |            |        |

# ILLNESS RECORD

| DATE | DIAGNOSIS | MEDICATION | DOCTOR |
|------|-----------|------------|--------|
|      |           |            |        |
|      |           |            |        |
|      |           |            |        |
|      |           |            |        |
|      |           |            |        |
|      |           |            |        |
|      |           |            |        |
|      |           |            |        |
|      |           |            |        |
|      |           |            |        |
|      |           |            |        |
|      |           |            |        |
|      |           |            |        |
|      |           |            |        |
|      |           |            |        |
|      |           |            |        |
|      |           |            |        |
|      |           |            |        |
|      |           |            |        |
|      |           |            |        |
|      |           |            |        |
|      |           |            |        |
|      |           |            |        |
|      |           |            |        |
|      |           |            |        |
|      |           |            |        |
|      |           |            |        |
|      |           |            |        |
|      |           |            |        |
|      |           |            |        |

# ILLNESS RECORD

| DATE | DIAGNOSIS | MEDICATION | DOCTOR |
|------|-----------|------------|--------|
|      |           |            |        |
|      |           |            |        |
|      |           |            |        |
|      |           |            |        |
|      |           |            |        |
|      |           |            |        |
|      |           |            |        |
|      |           |            |        |
|      |           |            |        |
|      |           |            |        |
|      |           |            |        |
|      |           |            |        |
|      |           |            |        |
|      |           |            |        |
|      |           |            |        |
|      |           |            |        |
|      |           |            |        |
|      |           |            |        |
|      |           |            |        |
|      |           |            |        |
|      |           |            |        |
|      |           |            |        |
|      |           |            |        |
|      |           |            |        |
|      |           |            |        |
|      |           |            |        |
|      |           |            |        |
|      |           |            |        |

# ILLNESS RECORD

| DATE | DIAGNOSIS | MEDICATION | DOCTOR |
|------|-----------|------------|--------|
|      |           |            |        |
|      |           |            |        |
|      |           |            |        |
|      |           |            |        |
|      |           |            |        |
|      |           |            |        |
|      |           |            |        |
|      |           |            |        |
|      |           |            |        |
|      |           |            |        |
|      |           |            |        |
|      |           |            |        |
|      |           |            |        |
|      |           |            |        |
|      |           |            |        |
|      |           |            |        |
|      |           |            |        |
|      |           |            |        |
|      |           |            |        |
|      |           |            |        |
|      |           |            |        |
|      |           |            |        |
|      |           |            |        |
|      |           |            |        |
|      |           |            |        |

# ILLNESS RECORD

| DATE | DIAGNOSIS | MEDICATION | DOCTOR |
|------|-----------|------------|--------|
|      |           |            |        |
|      |           |            |        |
|      |           |            |        |
|      |           |            |        |
|      |           |            |        |
|      |           |            |        |
|      |           |            |        |
|      |           |            |        |
|      |           |            |        |
|      |           |            |        |
|      |           |            |        |
|      |           |            |        |
|      |           |            |        |
|      |           |            |        |
|      |           |            |        |
|      |           |            |        |
|      |           |            |        |
|      |           |            |        |
|      |           |            |        |
|      |           |            |        |
|      |           |            |        |
|      |           |            |        |
|      |           |            |        |
|      |           |            |        |
|      |           |            |        |
|      |           |            |        |
|      |           |            |        |
|      |           |            |        |
|      |           |            |        |
|      |           |            |        |
|      |           |            |        |

# ILLNESS RECORD

| DATE | DIAGNOSIS | MEDICATION | DOCTOR |
|------|-----------|------------|--------|
|      |           |            |        |
|      |           |            |        |
|      |           |            |        |
|      |           |            |        |
|      |           |            |        |
|      |           |            |        |
|      |           |            |        |
|      |           |            |        |
|      |           |            |        |
|      |           |            |        |
|      |           |            |        |
|      |           |            |        |
|      |           |            |        |
|      |           |            |        |
|      |           |            |        |
|      |           |            |        |
|      |           |            |        |
|      |           |            |        |
|      |           |            |        |
|      |           |            |        |
|      |           |            |        |
|      |           |            |        |
|      |           |            |        |
|      |           |            |        |
|      |           |            |        |
|      |           |            |        |
|      |           |            |        |
|      |           |            |        |
|      |           |            |        |

# ILLNESS RECORD

| DATE | DIAGNOSIS | MEDICATION | DOCTOR |
|------|-----------|------------|--------|
|      |           |            |        |
|      |           |            |        |
|      |           |            |        |
|      |           |            |        |
|      |           |            |        |
|      |           |            |        |
|      |           |            |        |
|      |           |            |        |
|      |           |            |        |
|      |           |            |        |
|      |           |            |        |
|      |           |            |        |
|      |           |            |        |
|      |           |            |        |
|      |           |            |        |
|      |           |            |        |
|      |           |            |        |
|      |           |            |        |
|      |           |            |        |
|      |           |            |        |
|      |           |            |        |
|      |           |            |        |
|      |           |            |        |
|      |           |            |        |
|      |           |            |        |
|      |           |            |        |
|      |           |            |        |
|      |           |            |        |
|      |           |            |        |
|      |           |            |        |

# ILLNESS RECORD

| DATE | DIAGNOSIS | MEDICATION | DOCTOR |
|------|-----------|------------|--------|
|      |           |            |        |
|      |           |            |        |
|      |           |            |        |
|      |           |            |        |
|      |           |            |        |
|      |           |            |        |
|      |           |            |        |
|      |           |            |        |
|      |           |            |        |
|      |           |            |        |
|      |           |            |        |
|      |           |            |        |
|      |           |            |        |
|      |           |            |        |
|      |           |            |        |
|      |           |            |        |
|      |           |            |        |
|      |           |            |        |
|      |           |            |        |
|      |           |            |        |
|      |           |            |        |
|      |           |            |        |
|      |           |            |        |
|      |           |            |        |
|      |           |            |        |
|      |           |            |        |
|      |           |            |        |
|      |           |            |        |

# ILLNESS RECORD

| DATE | DIAGNOSIS | MEDICATION | DOCTOR |
|------|-----------|------------|--------|
|      |           |            |        |
|      |           |            |        |
|      |           |            |        |
|      |           |            |        |
|      |           |            |        |
|      |           |            |        |
|      |           |            |        |
|      |           |            |        |
|      |           |            |        |
|      |           |            |        |
|      |           |            |        |
|      |           |            |        |
|      |           |            |        |
|      |           |            |        |
|      |           |            |        |
|      |           |            |        |
|      |           |            |        |
|      |           |            |        |
|      |           |            |        |
|      |           |            |        |
|      |           |            |        |
|      |           |            |        |
|      |           |            |        |
|      |           |            |        |
|      |           |            |        |
|      |           |            |        |
|      |           |            |        |
|      |           |            |        |
|      |           |            |        |

# ILLNESS RECORD

| DATE | DIAGNOSIS | MEDICATION | DOCTOR |
|------|-----------|------------|--------|
|      |           |            |        |
|      |           |            |        |
|      |           |            |        |
|      |           |            |        |
|      |           |            |        |
|      |           |            |        |
|      |           |            |        |
|      |           |            |        |
|      |           |            |        |
|      |           |            |        |
|      |           |            |        |
|      |           |            |        |
|      |           |            |        |
|      |           |            |        |
|      |           |            |        |
|      |           |            |        |
|      |           |            |        |
|      |           |            |        |
|      |           |            |        |
|      |           |            |        |
|      |           |            |        |
|      |           |            |        |
|      |           |            |        |
|      |           |            |        |
|      |           |            |        |
|      |           |            |        |
|      |           |            |        |
|      |           |            |        |

# DOCTOR CONTACTS

| NAME | |
|---|---|
| PRACTICE | |
| CONTACT NUMBER | EMAIL |
| ADDRESS | |
| NOTES | |

| NAME | |
|---|---|
| PRACTICE | |
| CONTACT NUMBER | EMAIL |
| ADDRESS | |
| NOTES | |

| NAME | |
|---|---|
| PRACTICE | |
| CONTACT NUMBER | EMAIL |
| ADDRESS | |
| NOTES | |

| NAME | |
|---|---|
| PRACTICE | |
| CONTACT NUMBER | EMAIL |
| ADDRESS | |
| NOTES | |

# DOCTOR CONTACTS

| NAME | |
|---|---|
| PRACTICE | |
| CONTACT NUMBER | EMAIL |
| ADDRESS | |
| NOTES | |

| NAME | |
|---|---|
| PRACTICE | |
| CONTACT NUMBER | EMAIL |
| ADDRESS | |
| NOTES | |

| NAME | |
|---|---|
| PRACTICE | |
| CONTACT NUMBER | EMAIL |
| ADDRESS | |
| NOTES | |

| NAME | |
|---|---|
| PRACTICE | |
| CONTACT NUMBER | EMAIL |
| ADDRESS | |
| NOTES | |

# DOCTOR CONTACTS

| NAME | |
|------|---|
| PRACTICE | |
| CONTACT NUMBER | EMAIL |
| ADDRESS | |
| NOTES | |

| NAME | |
|------|---|
| PRACTICE | |
| CONTACT NUMBER | EMAIL |
| ADDRESS | |
| NOTES | |

| NAME | |
|------|---|
| PRACTICE | |
| CONTACT NUMBER | EMAIL |
| ADDRESS | |
| NOTES | |

| NAME | |
|------|---|
| PRACTICE | |
| CONTACT NUMBER | EMAIL |
| ADDRESS | |
| NOTES | |

# DOCTOR CONTACTS

| NAME | |
|------|---|
| PRACTICE | |
| CONTACT NUMBER | EMAIL |
| ADDRESS | |
| NOTES | |

| NAME | |
|------|---|
| PRACTICE | |
| CONTACT NUMBER | EMAIL |
| ADDRESS | |
| NOTES | |

| NAME | |
|------|---|
| PRACTICE | |
| CONTACT NUMBER | EMAIL |
| ADDRESS | |
| NOTES | |

| NAME | |
|------|---|
| PRACTICE | |
| CONTACT NUMBER | EMAIL |
| ADDRESS | |
| NOTES | |

# DOCTOR CONTACTS

| NAME | |
|---|---|
| PRACTICE | |
| CONTACT NUMBER | EMAIL |
| ADDRESS | |
| NOTES | |

| NAME | |
|---|---|
| PRACTICE | |
| CONTACT NUMBER | EMAIL |
| ADDRESS | |
| NOTES | |

| NAME | |
|---|---|
| PRACTICE | |
| CONTACT NUMBER | EMAIL |
| ADDRESS | |
| NOTES | |

| NAME | |
|---|---|
| PRACTICE | |
| CONTACT NUMBER | EMAIL |
| ADDRESS | |
| NOTES | |

# DOCTOR CONTACTS

| | |
|---|---|
| **NAME** | |
| **PRACTICE** | |
| **CONTACT NUMBER** | **EMAIL** |
| **ADDRESS** | |
| **NOTES** | |

| | |
|---|---|
| **NAME** | |
| **PRACTICE** | |
| **CONTACT NUMBER** | **EMAIL** |
| **ADDRESS** | |
| **NOTES** | |

| | |
|---|---|
| **NAME** | |
| **PRACTICE** | |
| **CONTACT NUMBER** | **EMAIL** |
| **ADDRESS** | |
| **NOTES** | |

| | |
|---|---|
| **NAME** | |
| **PRACTICE** | |
| **CONTACT NUMBER** | **EMAIL** |
| **ADDRESS** | |
| **NOTES** | |

# DOCTOR CONTACTS

| | |
|---|---|
| NAME | |
| PRACTICE | |
| CONTACT NUMBER | EMAIL |
| ADDRESS | |
| NOTES | |

| | |
|---|---|
| NAME | |
| PRACTICE | |
| CONTACT NUMBER | EMAIL |
| ADDRESS | |
| NOTES | |

| | |
|---|---|
| NAME | |
| PRACTICE | |
| CONTACT NUMBER | EMAIL |
| ADDRESS | |
| NOTES | |

| | |
|---|---|
| NAME | |
| PRACTICE | |
| CONTACT NUMBER | EMAIL |
| ADDRESS | |
| NOTES | |

# DOCTOR CONTACTS

| | |
|---|---|
| **NAME** | |
| **PRACTICE** | |
| **CONTACT NUMBER** | **EMAIL** |
| **ADDRESS** | |
| **NOTES** | |

| | |
|---|---|
| **NAME** | |
| **PRACTICE** | |
| **CONTACT NUMBER** | **EMAIL** |
| **ADDRESS** | |
| **NOTES** | |

| | |
|---|---|
| **NAME** | |
| **PRACTICE** | |
| **CONTACT NUMBER** | **EMAIL** |
| **ADDRESS** | |
| **NOTES** | |

| | |
|---|---|
| **NAME** | |
| **PRACTICE** | |
| **CONTACT NUMBER** | **EMAIL** |
| **ADDRESS** | |
| **NOTES** | |

# DOCTOR CONTACTS

| NAME | |
|---|---|
| PRACTICE | |
| CONTACT NUMBER | EMAIL |
| ADDRESS | |
| NOTES | |

| NAME | |
|---|---|
| PRACTICE | |
| CONTACT NUMBER | EMAIL |
| ADDRESS | |
| NOTES | |

| NAME | |
|---|---|
| PRACTICE | |
| CONTACT NUMBER | EMAIL |
| ADDRESS | |
| NOTES | |

| NAME | |
|---|---|
| PRACTICE | |
| CONTACT NUMBER | EMAIL |
| ADDRESS | |
| NOTES | |

# DOCTOR CONTACTS

| | |
|---|---|
| **NAME** | |
| **PRACTICE** | |
| **CONTACT NUMBER** | **EMAIL** |
| **ADDRESS** | |
| **NOTES** | |

| | |
|---|---|
| **NAME** | |
| **PRACTICE** | |
| **CONTACT NUMBER** | **EMAIL** |
| **ADDRESS** | |
| **NOTES** | |

| | |
|---|---|
| **NAME** | |
| **PRACTICE** | |
| **CONTACT NUMBER** | **EMAIL** |
| **ADDRESS** | |
| **NOTES** | |

| | |
|---|---|
| **NAME** | |
| **PRACTICE** | |
| **CONTACT NUMBER** | **EMAIL** |
| **ADDRESS** | |
| **NOTES** | |

# DENTAL RECORD

| DATE | DENTIST | TREATMENT | NOTES |
|------|---------|-----------|-------|
|  |  |  |  |
|  |  |  |  |
|  |  |  |  |
|  |  |  |  |
|  |  |  |  |
|  |  |  |  |
|  |  |  |  |
|  |  |  |  |
|  |  |  |  |
|  |  |  |  |
|  |  |  |  |
|  |  |  |  |
|  |  |  |  |
|  |  |  |  |
|  |  |  |  |
|  |  |  |  |
|  |  |  |  |
|  |  |  |  |
|  |  |  |  |
|  |  |  |  |
|  |  |  |  |
|  |  |  |  |
|  |  |  |  |
|  |  |  |  |
|  |  |  |  |
|  |  |  |  |
|  |  |  |  |
|  |  |  |  |
|  |  |  |  |
|  |  |  |  |
|  |  |  |  |
|  |  |  |  |

# DENTAL RECORD

| DATE | DENTIST | TREATMENT | NOTES |
|------|---------|-----------|-------|
|      |         |           |       |
|      |         |           |       |
|      |         |           |       |
|      |         |           |       |
|      |         |           |       |
|      |         |           |       |
|      |         |           |       |
|      |         |           |       |
|      |         |           |       |
|      |         |           |       |
|      |         |           |       |
|      |         |           |       |
|      |         |           |       |
|      |         |           |       |
|      |         |           |       |
|      |         |           |       |
|      |         |           |       |
|      |         |           |       |
|      |         |           |       |
|      |         |           |       |
|      |         |           |       |
|      |         |           |       |
|      |         |           |       |
|      |         |           |       |
|      |         |           |       |
|      |         |           |       |
|      |         |           |       |
|      |         |           |       |
|      |         |           |       |
|      |         |           |       |
|      |         |           |       |

# DENTAL RECORD

| DATE | DENTIST | TREATMENT | NOTES |
|------|---------|-----------|-------|
|      |         |           |       |
|      |         |           |       |
|      |         |           |       |
|      |         |           |       |
|      |         |           |       |
|      |         |           |       |
|      |         |           |       |
|      |         |           |       |
|      |         |           |       |
|      |         |           |       |
|      |         |           |       |
|      |         |           |       |
|      |         |           |       |
|      |         |           |       |
|      |         |           |       |
|      |         |           |       |
|      |         |           |       |
|      |         |           |       |
|      |         |           |       |
|      |         |           |       |
|      |         |           |       |
|      |         |           |       |
|      |         |           |       |
|      |         |           |       |
|      |         |           |       |
|      |         |           |       |
|      |         |           |       |
|      |         |           |       |
|      |         |           |       |
|      |         |           |       |
|      |         |           |       |

# DENTAL RECORD

| DATE | DENTIST | TREATMENT | NOTES |
|------|---------|-----------|-------|
|      |         |           |       |
|      |         |           |       |
|      |         |           |       |
|      |         |           |       |
|      |         |           |       |
|      |         |           |       |
|      |         |           |       |
|      |         |           |       |
|      |         |           |       |
|      |         |           |       |
|      |         |           |       |
|      |         |           |       |
|      |         |           |       |
|      |         |           |       |
|      |         |           |       |
|      |         |           |       |
|      |         |           |       |
|      |         |           |       |
|      |         |           |       |
|      |         |           |       |
|      |         |           |       |
|      |         |           |       |
|      |         |           |       |
|      |         |           |       |
|      |         |           |       |
|      |         |           |       |
|      |         |           |       |
|      |         |           |       |
|      |         |           |       |
|      |         |           |       |
|      |         |           |       |

# DENTAL RECORD

| DATE | DENTIST | TREATMENT | NOTES |
|------|---------|-----------|-------|
|      |         |           |       |
|      |         |           |       |
|      |         |           |       |
|      |         |           |       |
|      |         |           |       |
|      |         |           |       |
|      |         |           |       |
|      |         |           |       |
|      |         |           |       |
|      |         |           |       |
|      |         |           |       |
|      |         |           |       |
|      |         |           |       |
|      |         |           |       |
|      |         |           |       |
|      |         |           |       |
|      |         |           |       |
|      |         |           |       |
|      |         |           |       |
|      |         |           |       |
|      |         |           |       |
|      |         |           |       |
|      |         |           |       |
|      |         |           |       |
|      |         |           |       |
|      |         |           |       |
|      |         |           |       |
|      |         |           |       |
|      |         |           |       |
|      |         |           |       |
|      |         |           |       |

# DENTAL RECORD

| DATE | DENTIST | TREATMENT | NOTES |
|------|---------|-----------|-------|
|      |         |           |       |
|      |         |           |       |
|      |         |           |       |
|      |         |           |       |
|      |         |           |       |
|      |         |           |       |
|      |         |           |       |
|      |         |           |       |
|      |         |           |       |
|      |         |           |       |
|      |         |           |       |
|      |         |           |       |
|      |         |           |       |
|      |         |           |       |
|      |         |           |       |
|      |         |           |       |
|      |         |           |       |
|      |         |           |       |
|      |         |           |       |
|      |         |           |       |
|      |         |           |       |
|      |         |           |       |
|      |         |           |       |
|      |         |           |       |
|      |         |           |       |
|      |         |           |       |
|      |         |           |       |
|      |         |           |       |
|      |         |           |       |

# DENTAL RECORD

| DATE | DENTIST | TREATMENT | NOTES |
|------|---------|-----------|-------|
|      |         |           |       |
|      |         |           |       |
|      |         |           |       |
|      |         |           |       |
|      |         |           |       |
|      |         |           |       |
|      |         |           |       |
|      |         |           |       |
|      |         |           |       |
|      |         |           |       |
|      |         |           |       |
|      |         |           |       |
|      |         |           |       |
|      |         |           |       |
|      |         |           |       |
|      |         |           |       |
|      |         |           |       |
|      |         |           |       |
|      |         |           |       |
|      |         |           |       |
|      |         |           |       |
|      |         |           |       |
|      |         |           |       |
|      |         |           |       |
|      |         |           |       |
|      |         |           |       |
|      |         |           |       |
|      |         |           |       |

# DENTAL RECORD

| DATE | DENTIST | TREATMENT | NOTES |
|------|---------|-----------|-------|
| | | | |
| | | | |
| | | | |
| | | | |
| | | | |
| | | | |
| | | | |
| | | | |
| | | | |
| | | | |
| | | | |
| | | | |
| | | | |
| | | | |
| | | | |
| | | | |
| | | | |
| | | | |
| | | | |
| | | | |
| | | | |
| | | | |
| | | | |
| | | | |
| | | | |
| | | | |
| | | | |
| | | | |
| | | | |
| | | | |
| | | | |
| | | | |
| | | | |
| | | | |
| | | | |

# DENTAL RECORD

| DATE | DENTIST | TREATMENT | NOTES |
|------|---------|-----------|-------|
|      |         |           |       |
|      |         |           |       |
|      |         |           |       |
|      |         |           |       |
|      |         |           |       |
|      |         |           |       |
|      |         |           |       |
|      |         |           |       |
|      |         |           |       |
|      |         |           |       |
|      |         |           |       |
|      |         |           |       |
|      |         |           |       |
|      |         |           |       |
|      |         |           |       |
|      |         |           |       |
|      |         |           |       |
|      |         |           |       |
|      |         |           |       |
|      |         |           |       |
|      |         |           |       |
|      |         |           |       |
|      |         |           |       |
|      |         |           |       |
|      |         |           |       |
|      |         |           |       |
|      |         |           |       |
|      |         |           |       |
|      |         |           |       |
|      |         |           |       |
|      |         |           |       |

# DENTAL RECORD

| DATE | DENTIST | TREATMENT | NOTES |
|------|---------|-----------|-------|
|      |         |           |       |
|      |         |           |       |
|      |         |           |       |
|      |         |           |       |
|      |         |           |       |
|      |         |           |       |
|      |         |           |       |
|      |         |           |       |
|      |         |           |       |
|      |         |           |       |
|      |         |           |       |
|      |         |           |       |
|      |         |           |       |
|      |         |           |       |
|      |         |           |       |
|      |         |           |       |
|      |         |           |       |
|      |         |           |       |
|      |         |           |       |
|      |         |           |       |
|      |         |           |       |
|      |         |           |       |
|      |         |           |       |
|      |         |           |       |
|      |         |           |       |
|      |         |           |       |
|      |         |           |       |
|      |         |           |       |
|      |         |           |       |
|      |         |           |       |
|      |         |           |       |
|      |         |           |       |

# DOCTOR VISITS RECORD

| DATE | DOCTOR | REASON | NOTES |
|------|--------|--------|-------|
| | | | |
| | | | |
| | | | |
| | | | |
| | | | |
| | | | |
| | | | |
| | | | |
| | | | |
| | | | |
| | | | |
| | | | |
| | | | |
| | | | |
| | | | |
| | | | |
| | | | |
| | | | |
| | | | |
| | | | |
| | | | |
| | | | |
| | | | |
| | | | |
| | | | |
| | | | |
| | | | |
| | | | |

# DOCTOR VISITS RECORD

| DATE | DOCTOR | REASON | NOTES |
|------|--------|--------|-------|
|      |        |        |       |
|      |        |        |       |
|      |        |        |       |
|      |        |        |       |
|      |        |        |       |
|      |        |        |       |
|      |        |        |       |
|      |        |        |       |
|      |        |        |       |
|      |        |        |       |
|      |        |        |       |
|      |        |        |       |
|      |        |        |       |
|      |        |        |       |
|      |        |        |       |
|      |        |        |       |
|      |        |        |       |
|      |        |        |       |
|      |        |        |       |
|      |        |        |       |
|      |        |        |       |
|      |        |        |       |
|      |        |        |       |
|      |        |        |       |
|      |        |        |       |

# DOCTOR VISITS RECORD

| DATE | DOCTOR | REASON | NOTES |
|------|--------|--------|-------|
|      |        |        |       |
|      |        |        |       |
|      |        |        |       |
|      |        |        |       |
|      |        |        |       |
|      |        |        |       |
|      |        |        |       |
|      |        |        |       |
|      |        |        |       |
|      |        |        |       |
|      |        |        |       |
|      |        |        |       |
|      |        |        |       |
|      |        |        |       |
|      |        |        |       |
|      |        |        |       |
|      |        |        |       |
|      |        |        |       |
|      |        |        |       |
|      |        |        |       |
|      |        |        |       |
|      |        |        |       |
|      |        |        |       |
|      |        |        |       |
|      |        |        |       |
|      |        |        |       |
|      |        |        |       |
|      |        |        |       |
|      |        |        |       |
|      |        |        |       |

# DOCTOR VISITS RECORD

| DATE | DOCTOR | REASON | NOTES |
|------|--------|--------|-------|
|  |  |  |  |
|  |  |  |  |
|  |  |  |  |
|  |  |  |  |
|  |  |  |  |
|  |  |  |  |
|  |  |  |  |
|  |  |  |  |
|  |  |  |  |
|  |  |  |  |
|  |  |  |  |
|  |  |  |  |
|  |  |  |  |
|  |  |  |  |
|  |  |  |  |
|  |  |  |  |
|  |  |  |  |
|  |  |  |  |
|  |  |  |  |
|  |  |  |  |
|  |  |  |  |
|  |  |  |  |
|  |  |  |  |
|  |  |  |  |
|  |  |  |  |
|  |  |  |  |
|  |  |  |  |
|  |  |  |  |
|  |  |  |  |
|  |  |  |  |
|  |  |  |  |

# DOCTOR VISITS RECORD

| DATE | DOCTOR | REASON | NOTES |
|------|--------|--------|-------|
| | | | |
| | | | |
| | | | |
| | | | |
| | | | |
| | | | |
| | | | |
| | | | |
| | | | |
| | | | |
| | | | |
| | | | |
| | | | |
| | | | |
| | | | |
| | | | |
| | | | |
| | | | |
| | | | |
| | | | |
| | | | |
| | | | |
| | | | |
| | | | |
| | | | |
| | | | |
| | | | |
| | | | |
| | | | |
| | | | |

# DOCTOR VISITS RECORD

| DATE | DOCTOR | REASON | NOTES |
|------|--------|--------|-------|
|      |        |        |       |
|      |        |        |       |
|      |        |        |       |
|      |        |        |       |
|      |        |        |       |
|      |        |        |       |
|      |        |        |       |
|      |        |        |       |
|      |        |        |       |
|      |        |        |       |
|      |        |        |       |
|      |        |        |       |
|      |        |        |       |
|      |        |        |       |
|      |        |        |       |
|      |        |        |       |
|      |        |        |       |
|      |        |        |       |
|      |        |        |       |
|      |        |        |       |
|      |        |        |       |
|      |        |        |       |
|      |        |        |       |
|      |        |        |       |
|      |        |        |       |
|      |        |        |       |
|      |        |        |       |
|      |        |        |       |

# DOCTOR VISITS RECORD

| DATE | DOCTOR | REASON | NOTES |
|------|--------|--------|-------|
|      |        |        |       |
|      |        |        |       |
|      |        |        |       |
|      |        |        |       |
|      |        |        |       |
|      |        |        |       |
|      |        |        |       |
|      |        |        |       |
|      |        |        |       |
|      |        |        |       |
|      |        |        |       |
|      |        |        |       |
|      |        |        |       |
|      |        |        |       |
|      |        |        |       |
|      |        |        |       |
|      |        |        |       |
|      |        |        |       |
|      |        |        |       |
|      |        |        |       |
|      |        |        |       |
|      |        |        |       |
|      |        |        |       |
|      |        |        |       |
|      |        |        |       |
|      |        |        |       |
|      |        |        |       |
|      |        |        |       |
|      |        |        |       |

# DOCTOR VISITS RECORD

| DATE | DOCTOR | REASON | NOTES |
|------|--------|--------|-------|
|      |        |        |       |
|      |        |        |       |
|      |        |        |       |
|      |        |        |       |
|      |        |        |       |
|      |        |        |       |
|      |        |        |       |
|      |        |        |       |
|      |        |        |       |
|      |        |        |       |
|      |        |        |       |
|      |        |        |       |
|      |        |        |       |
|      |        |        |       |
|      |        |        |       |
|      |        |        |       |
|      |        |        |       |
|      |        |        |       |
|      |        |        |       |
|      |        |        |       |
|      |        |        |       |
|      |        |        |       |
|      |        |        |       |
|      |        |        |       |
|      |        |        |       |
|      |        |        |       |
|      |        |        |       |
|      |        |        |       |
|      |        |        |       |

# DOCTOR VISITS RECORD

| DATE | DOCTOR | REASON | NOTES |
|------|--------|--------|-------|
|      |        |        |       |
|      |        |        |       |
|      |        |        |       |
|      |        |        |       |
|      |        |        |       |
|      |        |        |       |
|      |        |        |       |
|      |        |        |       |
|      |        |        |       |
|      |        |        |       |
|      |        |        |       |
|      |        |        |       |
|      |        |        |       |
|      |        |        |       |
|      |        |        |       |
|      |        |        |       |
|      |        |        |       |
|      |        |        |       |
|      |        |        |       |
|      |        |        |       |
|      |        |        |       |
|      |        |        |       |
|      |        |        |       |
|      |        |        |       |
|      |        |        |       |
|      |        |        |       |
|      |        |        |       |
|      |        |        |       |
|      |        |        |       |

# DOCTOR VISITS RECORD

| DATE | DOCTOR | REASON | NOTES |
|------|--------|--------|-------|
|      |        |        |       |
|      |        |        |       |
|      |        |        |       |
|      |        |        |       |
|      |        |        |       |
|      |        |        |       |
|      |        |        |       |
|      |        |        |       |
|      |        |        |       |
|      |        |        |       |
|      |        |        |       |
|      |        |        |       |
|      |        |        |       |
|      |        |        |       |
|      |        |        |       |
|      |        |        |       |
|      |        |        |       |
|      |        |        |       |
|      |        |        |       |
|      |        |        |       |
|      |        |        |       |
|      |        |        |       |
|      |        |        |       |
|      |        |        |       |
|      |        |        |       |
|      |        |        |       |
|      |        |        |       |
|      |        |        |       |
|      |        |        |       |

# DOCTOR VISITS LOG

| | |
|---|---|
| **DATE** | **TIME** |
| **DOCTOR** | |
| **REASON FOR VISIT** | |
| **QUESTIONS TO ASK** | |
| **PRESCRIPTIONS** | |
| **NEXT VISIT** | |

| | |
|---|---|
| **DATE** | **TIME** |
| **DOCTOR** | |
| **REASON FOR VISIT** | |
| **QUESTIONS TO ASK** | |
| **PRESCRIPTIONS** | |
| **NEXT VISIT** | |

| | |
|---|---|
| **DATE** | **TIME** |
| **DOCTOR** | |
| **REASON FOR VISIT** | |
| **QUESTIONS TO ASK** | |
| **PRESCRIPTIONS** | |
| **NEXT VISIT** | |

# DOCTOR VISITS LOG

| DATE | | TIME | |
|------|--|------|--|
| DOCTOR | | | |
| REASON FOR VISIT | | | |
| QUESTIONS TO ASK | | | |
| PRESCRIPTIONS | | | |
| NEXT VISIT | | | |

| DATE | | TIME | |
|------|--|------|--|
| DOCTOR | | | |
| REASON FOR VISIT | | | |
| QUESTIONS TO ASK | | | |
| PRESCRIPTIONS | | | |
| NEXT VISIT | | | |

| DATE | | TIME | |
|------|--|------|--|
| DOCTOR | | | |
| REASON FOR VISIT | | | |
| QUESTIONS TO ASK | | | |
| PRESCRIPTIONS | | | |
| NEXT VISIT | | | |

# DOCTOR VISITS LOG

| | |
|---|---|
| **DATE** | **TIME** |
| **DOCTOR** | |
| **REASON FOR VISIT** | |
| **QUESTIONS TO ASK** | |
| **PRESCRIPTIONS** | |
| **NEXT VISIT** | |

| | |
|---|---|
| **DATE** | **TIME** |
| **DOCTOR** | |
| **REASON FOR VISIT** | |
| **QUESTIONS TO ASK** | |
| **PRESCRIPTIONS** | |
| **NEXT VISIT** | |

| | |
|---|---|
| **DATE** | **TIME** |
| **DOCTOR** | |
| **REASON FOR VISIT** | |
| **QUESTIONS TO ASK** | |
| **PRESCRIPTIONS** | |
| **NEXT VISIT** | |

# DOCTOR VISITS LOG

| DATE | | TIME | |
|---|---|---|---|
| DOCTOR | | | |
| REASON FOR VISIT | | | |
| QUESTIONS TO ASK | | | |
| PRESCRIPTIONS | | | |
| NEXT VISIT | | | |

| DATE | | TIME | |
|---|---|---|---|
| DOCTOR | | | |
| REASON FOR VISIT | | | |
| QUESTIONS TO ASK | | | |
| PRESCRIPTIONS | | | |
| NEXT VISIT | | | |

| DATE | | TIME | |
|---|---|---|---|
| DOCTOR | | | |
| REASON FOR VISIT | | | |
| QUESTIONS TO ASK | | | |
| PRESCRIPTIONS | | | |
| NEXT VISIT | | | |

# DOCTOR VISITS LOG

| DATE | | TIME | |
|---|---|---|---|
| DOCTOR | | | |
| REASON FOR VISIT | | | |
| QUESTIONS TO ASK | | | |
| PRESCRIPTIONS | | | |
| NEXT VISIT | | | |

| DATE | | TIME | |
|---|---|---|---|
| DOCTOR | | | |
| REASON FOR VISIT | | | |
| QUESTIONS TO ASK | | | |
| PRESCRIPTIONS | | | |
| NEXT VISIT | | | |

| DATE | | TIME | |
|---|---|---|---|
| DOCTOR | | | |
| REASON FOR VISIT | | | |
| QUESTIONS TO ASK | | | |
| PRESCRIPTIONS | | | |
| NEXT VISIT | | | |

# DOCTOR VISITS LOG

| DATE | | TIME | |
|------|--|------|--|
| **DOCTOR** | | | |
| **REASON FOR VISIT** | | | |
| **QUESTIONS TO ASK** | | | |
| **PRESCRIPTIONS** | | | |
| **NEXT VISIT** | | | |

| DATE | | TIME | |
|------|--|------|--|
| **DOCTOR** | | | |
| **REASON FOR VISIT** | | | |
| **QUESTIONS TO ASK** | | | |
| **PRESCRIPTIONS** | | | |
| **NEXT VISIT** | | | |

| DATE | | TIME | |
|------|--|------|--|
| **DOCTOR** | | | |
| **REASON FOR VISIT** | | | |
| **QUESTIONS TO ASK** | | | |
| **PRESCRIPTIONS** | | | |
| **NEXT VISIT** | | | |

# DOCTOR VISITS LOG

| DATE | | TIME | |
|---|---|---|---|
| DOCTOR | | | |
| REASON FOR VISIT | | | |
| QUESTIONS TO ASK | | | |
| PRESCRIPTIONS | | | |
| NEXT VISIT | | | |

| DATE | | TIME | |
|---|---|---|---|
| DOCTOR | | | |
| REASON FOR VISIT | | | |
| QUESTIONS TO ASK | | | |
| PRESCRIPTIONS | | | |
| NEXT VISIT | | | |

| DATE | | TIME | |
|---|---|---|---|
| DOCTOR | | | |
| REASON FOR VISIT | | | |
| QUESTIONS TO ASK | | | |
| PRESCRIPTIONS | | | |
| NEXT VISIT | | | |

# DOCTOR VISITS LOG

| DATE | | TIME | |
| --- | --- | --- | --- |
| DOCTOR | | | |
| REASON FOR VISIT | | | |
| QUESTIONS TO ASK | | | |
| PRESCRIPTIONS | | | |
| NEXT VISIT | | | |

| DATE | | TIME | |
| --- | --- | --- | --- |
| DOCTOR | | | |
| REASON FOR VISIT | | | |
| QUESTIONS TO ASK | | | |
| PRESCRIPTIONS | | | |
| NEXT VISIT | | | |

| DATE | | TIME | |
| --- | --- | --- | --- |
| DOCTOR | | | |
| REASON FOR VISIT | | | |
| QUESTIONS TO ASK | | | |
| PRESCRIPTIONS | | | |
| NEXT VISIT | | | |

# DOCTOR VISITS LOG

| DATE | | TIME | |
|------|------|------|------|
| DOCTOR | | | |
| REASON FOR VISIT | | | |
| QUESTIONS TO ASK | | | |
| PRESCRIPTIONS | | | |
| NEXT VISIT | | | |

| DATE | | TIME | |
|------|------|------|------|
| DOCTOR | | | |
| REASON FOR VISIT | | | |
| QUESTIONS TO ASK | | | |
| PRESCRIPTIONS | | | |
| NEXT VISIT | | | |

| DATE | | TIME | |
|------|------|------|------|
| DOCTOR | | | |
| REASON FOR VISIT | | | |
| QUESTIONS TO ASK | | | |
| PRESCRIPTIONS | | | |
| NEXT VISIT | | | |

# DOCTOR VISITS LOG

| DATE | | TIME | |
|------|--|------|--|
| DOCTOR | | | |
| REASON FOR VISIT | | | |
| QUESTIONS TO ASK | | | |
| PRESCRIPTIONS | | | |
| NEXT VISIT | | | |

| DATE | | TIME | |
|------|--|------|--|
| DOCTOR | | | |
| REASON FOR VISIT | | | |
| QUESTIONS TO ASK | | | |
| PRESCRIPTIONS | | | |
| NEXT VISIT | | | |

| DATE | | TIME | |
|------|--|------|--|
| DOCTOR | | | |
| REASON FOR VISIT | | | |
| QUESTIONS TO ASK | | | |
| PRESCRIPTIONS | | | |
| NEXT VISIT | | | |

# DOCTOR VISITS LOG

| DATE | | TIME | |
|------|--|------|--|
| DOCTOR | | | |
| REASON FOR VISIT | | | |
| QUESTIONS TO ASK | | | |
| PRESCRIPTIONS | | | |
| NEXT VISIT | | | |

| DATE | | TIME | |
|------|--|------|--|
| DOCTOR | | | |
| REASON FOR VISIT | | | |
| QUESTIONS TO ASK | | | |
| PRESCRIPTIONS | | | |
| NEXT VISIT | | | |

| DATE | | TIME | |
|------|--|------|--|
| DOCTOR | | | |
| REASON FOR VISIT | | | |
| QUESTIONS TO ASK | | | |
| PRESCRIPTIONS | | | |
| NEXT VISIT | | | |

# DOCTOR VISITS LOG

| DATE | | TIME | |
|------|--|------|--|
| DOCTOR | | | |
| REASON FOR VISIT | | | |
| QUESTIONS TO ASK | | | |
| PRESCRIPTIONS | | | |
| NEXT VISIT | | | |

| DATE | | TIME | |
|------|--|------|--|
| DOCTOR | | | |
| REASON FOR VISIT | | | |
| QUESTIONS TO ASK | | | |
| PRESCRIPTIONS | | | |
| NEXT VISIT | | | |

| DATE | | TIME | |
|------|--|------|--|
| DOCTOR | | | |
| REASON FOR VISIT | | | |
| QUESTIONS TO ASK | | | |
| PRESCRIPTIONS | | | |
| NEXT VISIT | | | |

# DOCTOR VISITS LOG

| DATE | | TIME | |
|------|--|------|--|
| DOCTOR | | | |
| REASON FOR VISIT | | | |
| QUESTIONS TO ASK | | | |
| PRESCRIPTIONS | | | |
| NEXT VISIT | | | |

| DATE | | TIME | |
|------|--|------|--|
| DOCTOR | | | |
| REASON FOR VISIT | | | |
| QUESTIONS TO ASK | | | |
| PRESCRIPTIONS | | | |
| NEXT VISIT | | | |

| DATE | | TIME | |
|------|--|------|--|
| DOCTOR | | | |
| REASON FOR VISIT | | | |
| QUESTIONS TO ASK | | | |
| PRESCRIPTIONS | | | |
| NEXT VISIT | | | |

# DOCTOR VISITS LOG

| DATE | | TIME | |
|------|------|------|------|
| DOCTOR | | | |
| REASON FOR VISIT | | | |
| QUESTIONS TO ASK | | | |
| PRESCRIPTIONS | | | |
| NEXT VISIT | | | |

| DATE | | TIME | |
|------|------|------|------|
| DOCTOR | | | |
| REASON FOR VISIT | | | |
| QUESTIONS TO ASK | | | |
| PRESCRIPTIONS | | | |
| NEXT VISIT | | | |

| DATE | | TIME | |
|------|------|------|------|
| DOCTOR | | | |
| REASON FOR VISIT | | | |
| QUESTIONS TO ASK | | | |
| PRESCRIPTIONS | | | |
| NEXT VISIT | | | |

# DOCTOR VISITS LOG

| DATE | | TIME | |
|---|---|---|---|
| DOCTOR | | | |
| REASON FOR VISIT | | | |
| QUESTIONS TO ASK | | | |
| PRESCRIPTIONS | | | |
| NEXT VISIT | | | |

| DATE | | TIME | |
|---|---|---|---|
| DOCTOR | | | |
| REASON FOR VISIT | | | |
| QUESTIONS TO ASK | | | |
| PRESCRIPTIONS | | | |
| NEXT VISIT | | | |

| DATE | | TIME | |
|---|---|---|---|
| DOCTOR | | | |
| REASON FOR VISIT | | | |
| QUESTIONS TO ASK | | | |
| PRESCRIPTIONS | | | |
| NEXT VISIT | | | |

# DOCTOR VISITS LOG

| DATE | | TIME | |
|---|---|---|---|
| DOCTOR | | | |
| REASON FOR VISIT | | | |
| QUESTIONS TO ASK | | | |
| PRESCRIPTIONS | | | |
| NEXT VISIT | | | |

| DATE | | TIME | |
|---|---|---|---|
| DOCTOR | | | |
| REASON FOR VISIT | | | |
| QUESTIONS TO ASK | | | |
| PRESCRIPTIONS | | | |
| NEXT VISIT | | | |

| DATE | | TIME | |
|---|---|---|---|
| DOCTOR | | | |
| REASON FOR VISIT | | | |
| QUESTIONS TO ASK | | | |
| PRESCRIPTIONS | | | |
| NEXT VISIT | | | |

# DOCTOR VISITS LOG

| DATE | | TIME | |
|---|---|---|---|
| DOCTOR | | | |
| REASON FOR VISIT | | | |
| QUESTIONS TO ASK | | | |
| PRESCRIPTIONS | | | |
| NEXT VISIT | | | |

| DATE | | TIME | |
|---|---|---|---|
| DOCTOR | | | |
| REASON FOR VISIT | | | |
| QUESTIONS TO ASK | | | |
| PRESCRIPTIONS | | | |
| NEXT VISIT | | | |

| DATE | | TIME | |
|---|---|---|---|
| DOCTOR | | | |
| REASON FOR VISIT | | | |
| QUESTIONS TO ASK | | | |
| PRESCRIPTIONS | | | |
| NEXT VISIT | | | |

# DOCTOR VISITS LOG

| DATE | | TIME | |
|---|---|---|---|
| **DOCTOR** | | | |
| **REASON FOR VISIT** | | | |
| **QUESTIONS TO ASK** | | | |
| **PRESCRIPTIONS** | | | |
| **NEXT VISIT** | | | |

| DATE | | TIME | |
|---|---|---|---|
| **DOCTOR** | | | |
| **REASON FOR VISIT** | | | |
| **QUESTIONS TO ASK** | | | |
| **PRESCRIPTIONS** | | | |
| **NEXT VISIT** | | | |

| DATE | | TIME | |
|---|---|---|---|
| **DOCTOR** | | | |
| **REASON FOR VISIT** | | | |
| **QUESTIONS TO ASK** | | | |
| **PRESCRIPTIONS** | | | |
| **NEXT VISIT** | | | |

# DOCTOR VISITS LOG

| DATE | | TIME | |
|---|---|---|---|
| DOCTOR | | | |
| REASON FOR VISIT | | | |
| QUESTIONS TO ASK | | | |
| PRESCRIPTIONS | | | |
| NEXT VISIT | | | |

| DATE | | TIME | |
|---|---|---|---|
| DOCTOR | | | |
| REASON FOR VISIT | | | |
| QUESTIONS TO ASK | | | |
| PRESCRIPTIONS | | | |
| NEXT VISIT | | | |

| DATE | | TIME | |
|---|---|---|---|
| DOCTOR | | | |
| REASON FOR VISIT | | | |
| QUESTIONS TO ASK | | | |
| PRESCRIPTIONS | | | |
| NEXT VISIT | | | |

# DOCTOR VISITS LOG

| DATE | | TIME | |
|---|---|---|---|
| DOCTOR | | | |
| REASON FOR VISIT | | | |
| QUESTIONS TO ASK | | | |
| PRESCRIPTIONS | | | |
| NEXT VISIT | | | |

| DATE | | TIME | |
|---|---|---|---|
| DOCTOR | | | |
| REASON FOR VISIT | | | |
| QUESTIONS TO ASK | | | |
| PRESCRIPTIONS | | | |
| NEXT VISIT | | | |

| DATE | | TIME | |
|---|---|---|---|
| DOCTOR | | | |
| REASON FOR VISIT | | | |
| QUESTIONS TO ASK | | | |
| PRESCRIPTIONS | | | |
| NEXT VISIT | | | |

# TEST RESULTS

| | |
|---|---|
| **DATE** | |
| **TEST** | |
| **DOCTOR** | |
| **REASON** | |
| **RESULT** | |

| | |
|---|---|
| **DATE** | |
| **TEST** | |
| **DOCTOR** | |
| **REASON** | |
| **RESULT** | |

| | |
|---|---|
| **DATE** | |
| **TEST** | |
| **DOCTOR** | |
| **REASON** | |
| **RESULT** | |

# TEST RESULTS

| DATE | |
|---|---|
| TEST | |
| DOCTOR | |
| REASON | |
| RESULT | |

| DATE | |
|---|---|
| TEST | |
| DOCTOR | |
| REASON | |
| RESULT | |

| DATE | |
|---|---|
| TEST | |
| DOCTOR | |
| REASON | |
| RESULT | |

# TEST RESULTS

| DATE | |
|---|---|
| TEST | |
| DOCTOR | |
| REASON | |
| RESULT | |

| DATE | |
|---|---|
| TEST | |
| DOCTOR | |
| REASON | |
| RESULT | |

| DATE | |
|---|---|
| TEST | |
| DOCTOR | |
| REASON | |
| RESULT | |

# TEST RESULTS

| | |
|---|---|
| DATE | |
| TEST | |
| DOCTOR | |
| REASON | |
| RESULT | |

| | |
|---|---|
| DATE | |
| TEST | |
| DOCTOR | |
| REASON | |
| RESULT | |

| | |
|---|---|
| DATE | |
| TEST | |
| DOCTOR | |
| REASON | |
| RESULT | |

# TEST RESULTS

| DATE | |
|---|---|
| TEST | |
| DOCTOR | |
| REASON | |
| RESULT | |

| DATE | |
|---|---|
| TEST | |
| DOCTOR | |
| REASON | |
| RESULT | |

| DATE | |
|---|---|
| TEST | |
| DOCTOR | |
| REASON | |
| RESULT | |

# TEST RESULTS

| DATE | |
| --- | --- |
| TEST | |
| DOCTOR | |
| REASON | |
| RESULT | |

| DATE | |
| --- | --- |
| TEST | |
| DOCTOR | |
| REASON | |
| RESULT | |

| DATE | |
| --- | --- |
| TEST | |
| DOCTOR | |
| REASON | |
| RESULT | |

# TEST RESULTS

| DATE | |
|---|---|
| TEST | |
| DOCTOR | |
| REASON | |
| RESULT | |

| DATE | |
|---|---|
| TEST | |
| DOCTOR | |
| REASON | |
| RESULT | |

| DATE | |
|---|---|
| TEST | |
| DOCTOR | |
| REASON | |
| RESULT | |

# TEST RESULTS

| DATE | |
|---|---|
| TEST | |
| DOCTOR | |
| REASON | |
| RESULT | |

| DATE | |
|---|---|
| TEST | |
| DOCTOR | |
| REASON | |
| RESULT | |

| DATE | |
|---|---|
| TEST | |
| DOCTOR | |
| REASON | |
| RESULT | |

# TEST RESULTS

| DATE | |
|------|------|
| TEST | |
| DOCTOR | |
| REASON | |
| RESULT | |

| DATE | |
|------|------|
| TEST | |
| DOCTOR | |
| REASON | |
| RESULT | |

| DATE | |
|------|------|
| TEST | |
| DOCTOR | |
| REASON | |
| RESULT | |

# TEST RESULTS

| DATE | |
|---|---|
| TEST | |
| DOCTOR | |
| REASON | |
| RESULT | |

| DATE | |
|---|---|
| TEST | |
| DOCTOR | |
| REASON | |
| RESULT | |

| DATE | |
|---|---|
| TEST | |
| DOCTOR | |
| REASON | |
| RESULT | |

# TEST RESULTS

| DATE | |
|---|---|
| TEST | |
| DOCTOR | |
| REASON | |
| RESULT | |

| DATE | |
|---|---|
| TEST | |
| DOCTOR | |
| REASON | |
| RESULT | |

| DATE | |
|---|---|
| TEST | |
| DOCTOR | |
| REASON | |
| RESULT | |

# TEST RESULTS

| DATE | |
|---|---|
| TEST | |
| DOCTOR | |
| REASON | |
| RESULT | |

| DATE | |
|---|---|
| TEST | |
| DOCTOR | |
| REASON | |
| RESULT | |

| DATE | |
|---|---|
| TEST | |
| DOCTOR | |
| REASON | |
| RESULT | |

# TEST RESULTS

| DATE | |
|---|---|
| TEST | |
| DOCTOR | |
| REASON | |
| RESULT | |

| DATE | |
|---|---|
| TEST | |
| DOCTOR | |
| REASON | |
| RESULT | |

| DATE | |
|---|---|
| TEST | |
| DOCTOR | |
| REASON | |
| RESULT | |

# TEST RESULTS

| DATE | |
|---|---|
| TEST | |
| DOCTOR | |
| REASON | |
| RESULT | |

| DATE | |
|---|---|
| TEST | |
| DOCTOR | |
| REASON | |
| RESULT | |

| DATE | |
|---|---|
| TEST | |
| DOCTOR | |
| REASON | |
| RESULT | |

# TEST RESULTS

| | |
|---|---|
| **DATE** | |
| **TEST** | |
| **DOCTOR** | |
| **REASON** | |
| **RESULT** | |

| | |
|---|---|
| **DATE** | |
| **TEST** | |
| **DOCTOR** | |
| **REASON** | |
| **RESULT** | |

| | |
|---|---|
| **DATE** | |
| **TEST** | |
| **DOCTOR** | |
| **REASON** | |
| **RESULT** | |

# TEST RESULTS

| DATE | |
| --- | --- |
| TEST | |
| DOCTOR | |
| REASON | |
| | |
| | |
| | |
| RESULT | |
| | |
| | |

| DATE | |
| --- | --- |
| TEST | |
| DOCTOR | |
| REASON | |
| | |
| | |
| | |
| RESULT | |
| | |
| | |

| DATE | |
| --- | --- |
| TEST | |
| DOCTOR | |
| REASON | |
| | |
| | |
| | |
| RESULT | |
| | |
| | |

# TEST RESULTS

| | |
|---|---|
| **DATE** | |
| **TEST** | |
| **DOCTOR** | |
| **REASON** | |
| **RESULT** | |

| | |
|---|---|
| **DATE** | |
| **TEST** | |
| **DOCTOR** | |
| **REASON** | |
| **RESULT** | |

| | |
|---|---|
| **DATE** | |
| **TEST** | |
| **DOCTOR** | |
| **REASON** | |
| **RESULT** | |

# TEST RESULTS

| DATE | |
|------|---|
| TEST | |
| DOCTOR | |
| REASON | |
| RESULT | |

| DATE | |
|------|---|
| TEST | |
| DOCTOR | |
| REASON | |
| RESULT | |

| DATE | |
|------|---|
| TEST | |
| DOCTOR | |
| REASON | |
| RESULT | |

# TEST RESULTS

| DATE | |
|---|---|
| TEST | |
| DOCTOR | |
| REASON | |
| RESULT | |

| DATE | |
|---|---|
| TEST | |
| DOCTOR | |
| REASON | |
| RESULT | |

| DATE | |
|---|---|
| TEST | |
| DOCTOR | |
| REASON | |
| RESULT | |

# TEST RESULTS

| DATE | |
|---|---|
| TEST | |
| DOCTOR | |
| REASON | |
| RESULT | |

| DATE | |
|---|---|
| TEST | |
| DOCTOR | |
| REASON | |
| RESULT | |

| DATE | |
|---|---|
| TEST | |
| DOCTOR | |
| REASON | |
| RESULT | |

# SURGICAL RECORD

| DATE | |
|---|---|
| SURGERY PERFORMED | |
| NAME OF DOCTOR | |
| NOTES | |

| DATE | |
|---|---|
| SURGERY PERFORMED | |
| NAME OF DOCTOR | |
| NOTES | |

| DATE | |
|---|---|
| SURGERY PERFORMED | |
| NAME OF DOCTOR | |
| NOTES | |

| DATE | |
|---|---|
| SURGERY PERFORMED | |
| NAME OF DOCTOR | |
| NOTES | |

# SURGICAL RECORD

| | |
|---|---|
| **DATE** | |
| **SURGERY PERFORMED** | |
| **NAME OF DOCTOR** | |
| **NOTES** | |

| | |
|---|---|
| **DATE** | |
| **SURGERY PERFORMED** | |
| **NAME OF DOCTOR** | |
| **NOTES** | |

| | |
|---|---|
| **DATE** | |
| **SURGERY PERFORMED** | |
| **NAME OF DOCTOR** | |
| **NOTES** | |

| | |
|---|---|
| **DATE** | |
| **SURGERY PERFORMED** | |
| **NAME OF DOCTOR** | |
| **NOTES** | |

# SURGICAL RECORD

| DATE | |
|------|---|
| SURGERY PERFORMED | |
| NAME OF DOCTOR | |
| NOTES | |

| DATE | |
|------|---|
| SURGERY PERFORMED | |
| NAME OF DOCTOR | |
| NOTES | |

| DATE | |
|------|---|
| SURGERY PERFORMED | |
| NAME OF DOCTOR | |
| NOTES | |

| DATE | |
|------|---|
| SURGERY PERFORMED | |
| NAME OF DOCTOR | |
| NOTES | |

# SURGICAL RECORD

| DATE | |
|------|--|
| SURGERY PERFORMED | |
| NAME OF DOCTOR | |
| NOTES | |

| DATE | |
|------|--|
| SURGERY PERFORMED | |
| NAME OF DOCTOR | |
| NOTES | |

| DATE | |
|------|--|
| SURGERY PERFORMED | |
| NAME OF DOCTOR | |
| NOTES | |

| DATE | |
|------|--|
| SURGERY PERFORMED | |
| NAME OF DOCTOR | |
| NOTES | |

# SURGICAL RECORD

| DATE | |
|---|---|
| SURGERY PERFORMED | |
| NAME OF DOCTOR | |
| NOTES | |

| DATE | |
|---|---|
| SURGERY PERFORMED | |
| NAME OF DOCTOR | |
| NOTES | |

| DATE | |
|---|---|
| SURGERY PERFORMED | |
| NAME OF DOCTOR | |
| NOTES | |

| DATE | |
|---|---|
| SURGERY PERFORMED | |
| NAME OF DOCTOR | |
| NOTES | |

# SURGICAL RECORD

| DATE | |
|---|---|
| SURGERY PERFORMED | |
| NAME OF DOCTOR | |
| NOTES | |

| DATE | |
|---|---|
| SURGERY PERFORMED | |
| NAME OF DOCTOR | |
| NOTES | |

| DATE | |
|---|---|
| SURGERY PERFORMED | |
| NAME OF DOCTOR | |
| NOTES | |

| DATE | |
|---|---|
| SURGERY PERFORMED | |
| NAME OF DOCTOR | |
| NOTES | |

# SURGICAL RECORD

| DATE | |
|------|--|
| SURGERY PERFORMED | |
| NAME OF DOCTOR | |
| NOTES | |

| DATE | |
|------|--|
| SURGERY PERFORMED | |
| NAME OF DOCTOR | |
| NOTES | |

| DATE | |
|------|--|
| SURGERY PERFORMED | |
| NAME OF DOCTOR | |
| NOTES | |

| DATE | |
|------|--|
| SURGERY PERFORMED | |
| NAME OF DOCTOR | |
| NOTES | |

# SURGICAL RECORD

| | |
|---|---|
| **DATE** | |
| **SURGERY PERFORMED** | |
| **NAME OF DOCTOR** | |
| **NOTES** | |

| | |
|---|---|
| **DATE** | |
| **SURGERY PERFORMED** | |
| **NAME OF DOCTOR** | |
| **NOTES** | |

| | |
|---|---|
| **DATE** | |
| **SURGERY PERFORMED** | |
| **NAME OF DOCTOR** | |
| **NOTES** | |

| | |
|---|---|
| **DATE** | |
| **SURGERY PERFORMED** | |
| **NAME OF DOCTOR** | |
| **NOTES** | |

# SURGICAL RECORD

| DATE | |
|---|---|
| SURGERY PERFORMED | |
| NAME OF DOCTOR | |
| NOTES | |

| DATE | |
|---|---|
| SURGERY PERFORMED | |
| NAME OF DOCTOR | |
| NOTES | |

| DATE | |
|---|---|
| SURGERY PERFORMED | |
| NAME OF DOCTOR | |
| NOTES | |

| DATE | |
|---|---|
| SURGERY PERFORMED | |
| NAME OF DOCTOR | |
| NOTES | |

# SURGICAL RECORD

| DATE | |
|---|---|
| SURGERY PERFORMED | |
| NAME OF DOCTOR | |
| NOTES | |

| DATE | |
|---|---|
| SURGERY PERFORMED | |
| NAME OF DOCTOR | |
| NOTES | |

| DATE | |
|---|---|
| SURGERY PERFORMED | |
| NAME OF DOCTOR | |
| NOTES | |

| DATE | |
|---|---|
| SURGERY PERFORMED | |
| NAME OF DOCTOR | |
| NOTES | |

# SURGICAL RECORD

| DATE | |
|---|---|
| SURGERY PERFORMED | |
| NAME OF DOCTOR | |
| NOTES | |

| DATE | |
|---|---|
| SURGERY PERFORMED | |
| NAME OF DOCTOR | |
| NOTES | |

| DATE | |
|---|---|
| SURGERY PERFORMED | |
| NAME OF DOCTOR | |
| NOTES | |

| DATE | |
|---|---|
| SURGERY PERFORMED | |
| NAME OF DOCTOR | |
| NOTES | |

# SURGICAL RECORD

| | |
|---|---|
| **DATE** | |
| **SURGERY PERFORMED** | |
| **NAME OF DOCTOR** | |
| **NOTES** | |

| | |
|---|---|
| **DATE** | |
| **SURGERY PERFORMED** | |
| **NAME OF DOCTOR** | |
| **NOTES** | |

| | |
|---|---|
| **DATE** | |
| **SURGERY PERFORMED** | |
| **NAME OF DOCTOR** | |
| **NOTES** | |

| | |
|---|---|
| **DATE** | |
| **SURGERY PERFORMED** | |
| **NAME OF DOCTOR** | |
| **NOTES** | |

# SURGICAL RECORD

| DATE | |
| --- | --- |
| SURGERY PERFORMED | |
| NAME OF DOCTOR | |
| NOTES | |

| DATE | |
| --- | --- |
| SURGERY PERFORMED | |
| NAME OF DOCTOR | |
| NOTES | |

| DATE | |
| --- | --- |
| SURGERY PERFORMED | |
| NAME OF DOCTOR | |
| NOTES | |

| DATE | |
| --- | --- |
| SURGERY PERFORMED | |
| NAME OF DOCTOR | |
| NOTES | |

# SURGICAL RECORD

| DATE | |
|---|---|
| SURGERY PERFORMED | |
| NAME OF DOCTOR | |
| NOTES | |

| DATE | |
|---|---|
| SURGERY PERFORMED | |
| NAME OF DOCTOR | |
| NOTES | |

| DATE | |
|---|---|
| SURGERY PERFORMED | |
| NAME OF DOCTOR | |
| NOTES | |

| DATE | |
|---|---|
| SURGERY PERFORMED | |
| NAME OF DOCTOR | |
| NOTES | |

# SURGICAL RECORD

| DATE | |
|---|---|
| SURGERY PERFORMED | |
| NAME OF DOCTOR | |
| NOTES | |

| DATE | |
|---|---|
| SURGERY PERFORMED | |
| NAME OF DOCTOR | |
| NOTES | |

| DATE | |
|---|---|
| SURGERY PERFORMED | |
| NAME OF DOCTOR | |
| NOTES | |

| DATE | |
|---|---|
| SURGERY PERFORMED | |
| NAME OF DOCTOR | |
| NOTES | |

# SURGICAL RECORD

| DATE | |
|---|---|
| SURGERY PERFORMED | |
| NAME OF DOCTOR | |
| NOTES | |

| DATE | |
|---|---|
| SURGERY PERFORMED | |
| NAME OF DOCTOR | |
| NOTES | |

| DATE | |
|---|---|
| SURGERY PERFORMED | |
| NAME OF DOCTOR | |
| NOTES | |

| DATE | |
|---|---|
| SURGERY PERFORMED | |
| NAME OF DOCTOR | |
| NOTES | |

# SURGICAL RECORD

| DATE | |
|---|---|
| **SURGERY PERFORMED** | |
| **NAME OF DOCTOR** | |
| **NOTES** | |

| DATE | |
|---|---|
| **SURGERY PERFORMED** | |
| **NAME OF DOCTOR** | |
| **NOTES** | |

| DATE | |
|---|---|
| **SURGERY PERFORMED** | |
| **NAME OF DOCTOR** | |
| **NOTES** | |

| DATE | |
|---|---|
| **SURGERY PERFORMED** | |
| **NAME OF DOCTOR** | |
| **NOTES** | |

# SURGICAL RECORD

| DATE | |
| --- | --- |
| SURGERY PERFORMED | |
| NAME OF DOCTOR | |
| NOTES | |

| DATE | |
| --- | --- |
| SURGERY PERFORMED | |
| NAME OF DOCTOR | |
| NOTES | |

| DATE | |
| --- | --- |
| SURGERY PERFORMED | |
| NAME OF DOCTOR | |
| NOTES | |

| DATE | |
| --- | --- |
| SURGERY PERFORMED | |
| NAME OF DOCTOR | |
| NOTES | |

# SURGICAL RECORD

| DATE | |
|---|---|
| SURGERY PERFORMED | |
| NAME OF DOCTOR | |
| NOTES | |

| DATE | |
|---|---|
| SURGERY PERFORMED | |
| NAME OF DOCTOR | |
| NOTES | |

| DATE | |
|---|---|
| SURGERY PERFORMED | |
| NAME OF DOCTOR | |
| NOTES | |

| DATE | |
|---|---|
| SURGERY PERFORMED | |
| NAME OF DOCTOR | |
| NOTES | |

# SURGICAL RECORD

| DATE | |
|---|---|
| SURGERY PERFORMED | |
| NAME OF DOCTOR | |
| NOTES | |

| DATE | |
|---|---|
| SURGERY PERFORMED | |
| NAME OF DOCTOR | |
| NOTES | |

| DATE | |
|---|---|
| SURGERY PERFORMED | |
| NAME OF DOCTOR | |
| NOTES | |

| DATE | |
|---|---|
| SURGERY PERFORMED | |
| NAME OF DOCTOR | |
| NOTES | |

# NOTES

# NOTES

# NOTES

# NOTES

# NOTES

# NOTES

# NOTES

# NOTES

# NOTES

# NOTES

Made in the USA
Coppell, TX
28 August 2023